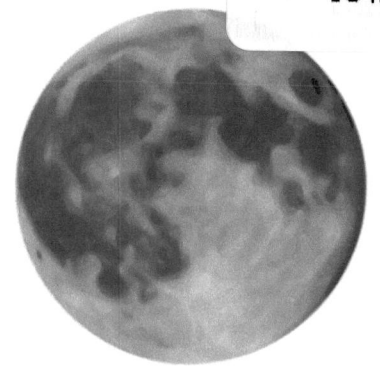

Slowness Gives Wholeness

Decelerating into Transformation

ANTHONY JAMES CANELO

ISBN: 1490302190

ISBN 13: 9781490302195

Library of Congress Control Number: 2013910236

CreateSpace Independent Publishing Platform
North Charleston, South Carolina

OTHER BOOKS BY ANTHONY CANELO

The Nature Pyramid

The Seven Fundamentals of Longevity

Marriage, Incarceration, Death, Religion, and Patience

Sleep: The Great Medicine

Creationships

Folk Remedies For The Modern Age

The Complete Compact Guide to Disaster Survival

Revival of the Fittest: The Prime Material for Human Health and Wisdom

The Revival of the Fittest: A Manual to Change the World

Self Determination: The Strategy to Master Addiction in America

TABLE OF CONTENTS

LAO TZU

"If you want to shrink something, you must first allow it to expand. If you want to get rid of something, you must first allow it to flourish. If you want to take something, you must first allow it to be given. This is called the subtler perception of the way things are. The soft overcomes the hard. The slow overcomes the fast. Let your workings remain a mystery. Just show people the results."

A MODERN VERSION OF THE 23RD PSALM

THE LORD is my Pace

setter - I shall not rush.

He makes me stop for quiet intervals,

He provides me with images of stillness

which restore my serenity,

He leads me in ways of efficiency

through calmness of mind,

And his guidance is peace.

Even though I have a great many things to

accomplish each day, I will not fret,

For his presence is here,

His timelessness, His all-importance,

will keep me in balance

He prepares refreshment and renewal

in the midst of my activity,

By anointing my mind with His oils of tranquility,

My cup of joyous energy overflows.

Truly, harmony and effectiveness

shall be the fruits of my hours,

For I shall walk in the Pace of my Lord

And dwell in His House forever.

BY

TOKIO MEGASHIA

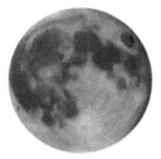

The Old Man
And The Orchard

In an ancient valley, in a round house, on the front of an old banana orchard, lived an old wise man. He sat alone in his lemon wood chair, listening for his visitors to arrive. On arrival, his new visitor took an eager seat in front of this old wise man, with fluttering eyes and a flashy broad grin. The old wise man imparted a polite greeting to him, then instructed him as to the rules of the game that they were going to play.

When the rules were made clear, they focused in stillness and quiet for a brief time.

The young visitor began to perspire from his forehead.

The old wise man looked beyond the young man, waiting, completely still.

In the wise man's outstretched palm there was a large, polished, black diamond.

It was for the taking, provided that the young man was deft enough to snatch it out of his gentle wrinkled palm. If so, the large diamond and the orchard would be his forever.

In the blink of an eye, the wise man's palm collapsed, retracting swiftly into his pocket. The game was over. The young man, though sullen, made his polite exit with a smile and was not seen again.

Though time had ravaged the edifice of this old, wise man, his super keen reflexes were beyond reckoning.

There came many visitors to his humble home. All of them were eager to acquire the orchard, hoping to grasp a heavy, shiny piece of forever in the process. There were those virtuous guests of the home, and then there were those manipulative, clever folk who visited him. None would steal the black diamond from his palm.

There came one day a wise young warrior on horseback from an unknown territory in the west who circled the ancient valley four times prior to receiving word of the bizarre orchard lottery.

In the moment he understood, this man unsaddled himself beside a quiet river to contemplate such an incredible opportunity within his dreams.

When six days had passed the young man approached the round home on horseback. He tied his horse to a large maple tree. He entered the old man's home in a calculated and polite fashion.

The young man understood the rules of the game several days prior to the old man who instructed him from his seat. In the moments that the old man spoke, the young man hit upon a stunning and unique observation: the wise man could not see. He was blind.

This he noticed because the old man always seemed to gaze beyond him, never in his eye. Then, within the last moments of instruction, the young man cleverly disrobed. It was understood that the old wise man reacted not from visual impulse, but from an auditory impulse.

So he sat there with the old wise man, completely nude, engaged in the sweet and timeless art of concentration.

The old man looked beyond him, unmoved. Five hours passed and nobody moved. In the next five hours, the young warrior's wrist rotated upwards, ever so slowly and ever so quietly. The setting sun brought dazzling color and hue through the room. The window upon the wall brought a gentle wind over the old man.

The singing of birds, the laughter of children, these things did not go by unnoticed, nor unappreciated.

Many hours into the night did the young man sit with this old and wise man. When the morning dew began to form on the young man's eye lashes, his hand was relaxed and open, his arm was halfway extended toward the shiny, black diamond. Several more long hours passed.

At noon, lunch was served to the small children. The understated poise of the old man went unchanged.

By four o'clock, the young man's palm began to cast a light shadow over the old man's palm. All the time, he was getting closer and closer and closer.

At dawn, in a moment of profound peace, the young man's hand was nearly on the diamond. There, the old man lifted his chin. He proudly procured the black diamond from his left palm by his right two fingers and placed it into the young man's outstretched hand.

The old and wise man said, "I have observed within you the character, patience, and mind of a true wise man. You are a man who is fit to tend to the duties of my beloved orchard. You are a man who can patiently watch the beautiful ripening of our fruit, so far into spring. Bless you and your family on this immortal and enchanted evening! My diamond and my land now are yours!"

Then the smiling old man sat back in his chair, wiped a few tears from his clear blue eyes, and vanished into the great unknown.

-Anthony James Canelo

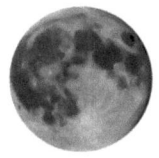

Introduction

'*Slowness Gives Wholeness*' was born out of my personal journey through life. I was born in the month of the lion, on the fifth hour of the sixth day. I have owned and managed two businesses, written four books, and lived in six states. I am twenty-six years old. I was born a fast mover. Privately, my mistakes and failures amount equally.

However, I never tire of trying. I am intoxicated by the rhythm of evolution. A wise man once said to me, "If you want to learn something, teach it." For the most part, he was correct.

Just for the record, I take slow, long, barefoot walks in my local park. If I see you there, I will try not to run you over.

During my walks, what I have observed is that nature is moving at a much slower and more deliberate pace. Nature's most industrious creatures can hardly be seen. Nature's fastest creatures are often the quietest. Imagine if children were taught to behave deliberately and patiently, following their standard "Birds & The Bees" chat. We would all be living in a vastly different world.

This is a health book. It is a message about the natural rhythm of life. Slowness really does bring wholeness. What does sleeping bring? Sleep brings wholeness and inner peace. What do companionship and a connection to nature bring? Each bring stillness and joy. What does exercise give? Exercise gives patience. What does breathing give? Breathing gives whole-mindedness and calmness. What does a wholesome diet provide? A wholesome diet provides health and wholeness. What about hydration? What about a self self-loving attitude?

If you do not believe in your own power to advance yourself, you have opened the wrong book.

My longevity Pyramid boils human health down to seven essentials, a blueprint for success. Most essential is breathing, followed by sleeping, then drinking, attitude, eating, exercise, and a connection to nature. These days it is easy to get trapped into one or two essentials, ignoring the other metabolic and energetic necessities of existence. If you are aspiring to be healthy and healed, you are aspiring to this blue print. In my last book, 'The Seven Fundamentals of Longevity", I discuss the architecture of the longevity pyramid. 'Slowness Gives Wholeness', the book you now have in your hands, is my Longevity Pyramid, re- conceptualized

In the best way I know how, I am going to create refreshing ways for you to touch the whole. That being the vast, unseen continuum; the heart; the observer; or the great, deep rhythm of stillness.

Herein lay some viable options for you to use to explore time, nature, rhythm, and energy. "A master of rhythm is a master of energy." Another wise old man told me that one. I think he was absolutely onto something. "'What?" you may ask?

Together, let us take our time and find out. When we are centered, we explore ultimate mobility for change. If you are standing still in the center of a field, searching for three hundred and sixty degrees of potential directions, you have given yourself the most intelligent quantity of options. Life is like that.

Do take your time as you read this book. I hope that, as you do, your options become more centered, more balanced, more unlimited. May you get to where you are going for slower or for worse.

Anthony James Canelo

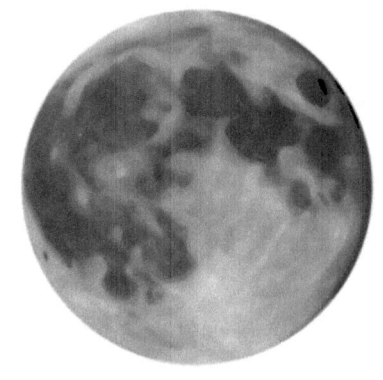

Breathing

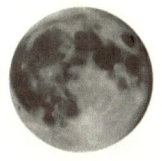

Your Breath is Golden

No material thing, no secret doctrine, no herb, no capsule, no vitamin, no elixir, no plant, no chant, no mantra, nor ritual or guru, nor woman or man, nor wine or spirits can help to teach you how to live with an attitude of pure wisdom and harmony more effectively than your own breath.

Focus on a slow, deep, long breath now.

Place your hand on your heart, wrist, or other pulse point. Gauge your body's rhythm for a moment. Now, focus on taking forty slow, long, deep breaths. By all means, take your time. Observe your natural body rhythm. Is your pulse beating slower? Are you more relaxed?

How much energy did you save? Does it matter if you cannot measure it?

Observe your emotional state. Can you feel a new tranquility, deep calmness, or slowness? Insofar as emotional release is concerned, I know of no greater tool than a dedicated routine of focused breathing.

Let us examine the focused breathing practices that help us to *slow down.* They include the slow, blinking breath; the blind bumblebee breath; "playing the horn;" and "singing a simple song."

SLOW BREATHING AND SLOW BLINKING

Imagine you are waking from the most delightful dream. Ever so gently, begin to raise your eyelids. This action, if repeated very slowly, has an instant hypnotic effect.

Now, in a pure moment of relaxation, slowly breathe in. When you have filled your lungs, count backward from four, and then—ever so gently, ever so slowly—breathe out. You will slowly lower your heart rate and blood pressure while you improve brain and liver circulation by this simple, repeated action.

Now we will practice them together.

FROM THE DARKNESS COMES THE LIGHT

As you inhale, gently close your eyes while imagining vital energy and wisdom filling you.

Whenever you pause to reflect or think, you will likely close your eyes to avoid distraction. It is a reflex. We do this because, physiologically, this brief period of darkness greatly aids the cognitive process. Is this your first time reading this book? Thus far, how many times have you blinked slowly? Remember, your eyes are an important part of your brain.

Following your deep inhale and contemplative slow blink, retain the breath for four seconds, and begin to slowly exhale, returning the measure of your wisdom and vital energy to the light.

As your eyelids open, visualize yourself in a different reality, with a new understanding. We all have eyelids, you know. Most people have just forgotten how to use them. The interplay of darkness and light plays a critical role in the functioning of mental ability, eye health, and hormone health.

You may repeat this process for five minutes at least five times a day to experience the wonderful benefits of darkness and light. Memorize the following instructions, then repeat them to yourself prior to your practice, if you wish: *I awaken from my dream. I inhale with my contemplative blink. In my darkness, I hold my understanding. Now, I slowly exhale into the light of new understanding.*

THE BLIND
BUMBLEBEE BREATH

If you need to center and calm yourself quickly, this is the breath for you. Begin by tapping yourself on the top of your head for about ninety seconds as you focus intently on breathing slowly. Is anybody home?

This whole performance will help you become grounded in your natural rhythm of breathing. If you choose to rub your stomach, you may do so. After ninety seconds, place two fingers over each eye, your middle and pointer, and close the holes in your ears with your thumbs. Your eyes should be closed. You are engaging the element of sensory deprivation before starting the blind bumblebee breath.

Now inhale and slowly buzz or hum at a very low volume, like a bumblebee. You should feel a sound vibration moving into your stomach, chest, head, or throat. This vibration has an astonishingly profound, hypnotic effect. Try to learn how to focus this vibrational wave toward any part of your body that needs healing. If you feel confident in moving sound, you can experience its tremendous healing powers.

An excellent time to practice the blind bumblebee breath is in the bathroom at your job or before sleeping. It will help to tranquilize your brain and alleviate stress.

PLAYING THE HORN

Some of the best breathers I know play the trumpet. It might sound like a troubling amount of effort; however, there are proven benefits to playing instruments like the trumpet, flute, saxophone, tuba, or clarinet that go way beyond the respiratory system.

Did you know that musicians in ancient Egypt knew how to play the trumpet? As an emotional outlet and exercise in ear-hand coordination, playing the horn nourishes the creative potential of any human being with a good set of lungs and ears.

I strongly suggest that you begin your adventure on the horn by sampling the music of Miles Davis. In my opinion, Miles Davis was a grand master in the art of musical stillness. Beginners should find it easy to listen to, appreciate, and imitate a few of Miles Davis's songs. He had an incredible tone and used silence effectively. Carlos Santana once remarked, "Listening to Miles Davis helped me learn how to use space and silence."

For young readers, I recommend the albums *Kind of Blue* or *Doo Bop. Older* listeners might try *Kind of Blue, Miles Ahead,* or *Sketches of Spain.*

For enjoyment, I recommend listening to the music of Nils Frahm. His popular albums are named 'Screws', 'Felt', 'Electric Piano', and 'The Bells'. Nils Frahm is a grand master of stillness, an unmistakable musical prodigy. Not many people can create a four minute rhapsody using a single note on the piano. I also suggest you listen to the 'Hemi Sync' collection, by Monroe

Products. These albums utilize an ingenious patented technology designed to balance and refocus the brain. This technology works astonishingly well. A full playlist featuring my favorite relaxing tunes is available on my website, www.PhoenixInstituteOnline.com.

SLOW SINGING

One of the beautiful things about the music of Miles Davis is that he rarely used a vibrato. Miles learned to take his time on the horn, playing mostly flat tones that are rich and simple.

Singing in a simple way allows you to inhale slowly and exhale with dynamic integrity. Selecting a mellow, simple song to sing can ease the mind, slow your heart rate, and bring joy into your life. I recommend you sing a simple song every day.

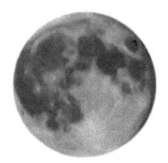

#1 Health Fundamental: Breathing

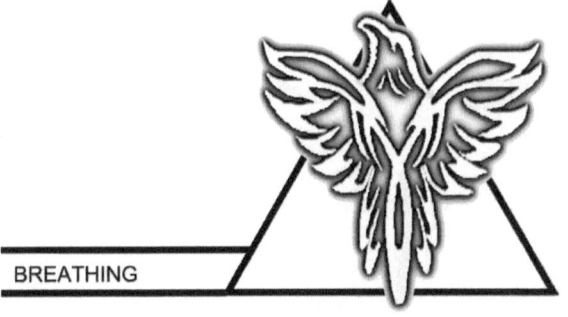

BREATHING

You can determine the degree to which someone feels comfortable around one or more persons by his or her shortness of breath. If a scientist were to conduct an experiment on a large group of Wall Street day traders in order to gauge how each person feels about a particular company, he would merely need to attach breath monitors to their lapels and monitor the rise and fall of carbon dioxide in the trading rooms. Breathing is that powerful.

At the Phoenix Institute, I was once introduced to a young man in his early twenties with severe autism. His mother severely doubted whether I could administer an ionic foot bath to him for any significant period of time, because all day he constantly moved and could not seem to get control of himself. I felt an enormous amount of compassion for the young man because I, too, know what it's like not to be in control of one's faculties. I knew what to do.

I observed his mother insisting that he relax, to no avail. She went outside to make a long phone call. I stayed with him. I made eye contact with him, politely grinned, and began a long series of deep, powerful breaths. I observed that the young man showed no interest in following any instructions. If I breathed, he breathed. If I spoke, he spoke. If I stood up, he stood up. He was a great imitator. Later, I learned he was a musical savant, an incredibly talented drummer.

I led him through a series of powerful breaths, then a series of short, slow breaths, followed by a series of limbic exhales, followed by a series of powerful athletic breaths, followed by a series of alternate nostril breaths, followed by a series of blind bumblebee breaths, followed by a series of fire breaths, followed by a series of quick exhales, followed by a series of slow exhales. Within the span of twenty minutes, he and I were like two young dragons. He kept his feet still in the foot bath the entire time.

I have never met anyone who could follow my instructions perfectly, without being taught. His body, like mine, hungered for atmosphere. He was a sensitive young man; he could feel that primal need for air. Toward the end, I found the change in his behavior entirely obvious. When his mother returned, I made sure she saw us breathing, and her son felt proud to show her what he learned. He looked calm, collected, and finally attentive to people. To say his mother looked shocked would be an understatement. Both felt happy to have visited me. My doors are always open to them.

I instructed his mother to stop using the words "relax," "calm down," or, "be quiet." Instead, I suggested she replace those words with, "Breathe, breathe. Good job;" or, "You can do it. Breathe slowly;" and, "Very good. Breathe." This seemed to help their relationship tremendously.

I also instructed her to breathe ten to thirty minutes a day with him while following several of the techniques I have written in my third book, *The Seven Fundamentals of Longevity & the Holistic Health Pyramid.*

You do not need a family member who is autistic to benefit from the instruction I gave to her. That day I urged her to keep switching techniques so that this nice, young man could feel engaged and remain on the right side—or imaginative side—of his brain, where he lived most of the time.

I would make the same recommendation to anyone else. Keep alternating techniques during your breathing practice to engage the right side of your brain. By all means, you can blow out some steam every once in a while, just like the dragons who dwell at the Phoenix Institute.

How big is the medicine of the breath? In our society, we tend to do important things too quickly, and unimportant things too slowly. Make room in your life for fulfillment. Take your time and rediscover the breath of life.

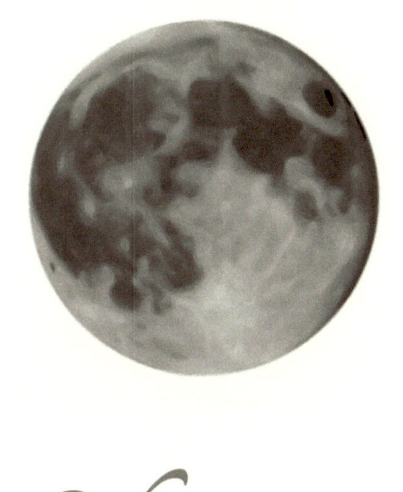

Sleeping

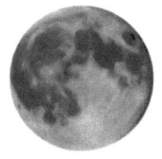

The Nocturnal Shift

Do you know the feeling of lying down to go to sleep at night, dreaming long and sweetly, and rising up in the total peace of physical restoration? Perhaps you last sampled this nocturnal bliss—this divine rest—in childhood. Many of us think of such rest as the hallmark of our earlier years, and that waking up with a vivacious spirit and rested body is solely the distinction of youth. It's just not true.

I think true love is the fresh beginning of every new day, a feeling that inspires a state of wonder in most children. True love helps us remember that every moment is actually authentic and filled with possibility, despite what is happening in our lives. That singular feeling exists as a remote dream in the minds of most adults and its solitary magic and softness are our lost treasures. Nonetheless, we can experience it during a beautiful sunrise, when we are paying attention. In the final analysis, it appears that if you live an utterly busy life, like a chicken with its head sliced off, your sleep will reflect exactly that.

VALUE OF ATTITUDE

Rest assured that this, too, will change. If you can meditate, you have the ability to change your attitude. Through meditation, you can improve the functioning of your brain. If you strive to improve your wellbeing and health, you can have no better meditative focus than an abundance of deep, healing rest. Impeccable attitude, deep breathing, and quality sleep are all bottom-line fundamentals of health. Sleep engages all three of these fundamentals at their highest potential. "How convenient!" you may say. Indeed.

We are only beginning to understand the revitalizing power of attitude. The demand for this type of knowledge has increased dramatically due to spiritual confusion. Many claim to have all the answers; however, the best teachers among us cannot transmit experiential knowledge. Experience lies at the heart of learning. This is why I strongly suggest you meditate for thirty minutes at night as an ideal beginning to your own practice of mindfulness.

Healing your body with your attitude is challenging, yet possible. If you want to heal your body and calm your mind, consider the following instructions.

SLEEPING IS HEALING

According to the human body, sleeping *is* healing. When you arrive at your bed tonight, blindfold yourself, lie down, and contemplate "sleeping is healing" for a few minutes as you would any other important issue in your life.

As you contemplate, breathe slowly. Ask yourself how much you are willing to heal your body. Does the amount equal the amount of tiredness you feel right now? Do you feel uncertain of how well you will sleep, yet certain *you can and deserve to be restored?*

Now, slowly move your focus into your body while maintaining a relaxed state of mind. When you're ready, practice patience within your body. In other words, create an attitude of patience that you can feel through focus and imagination. Do this for fifteen minutes as you continue to breathe slowly. You are preparing your spirit for its final, conscious job of the day.

After you have thoroughly embodied your state of patience, bring that same focus to your spirit. During the day, your spirit resides inside your body. At night, your energy body expands and your spirit journeys elsewhere. The spirit (or the deeper mind) is your dreamer and is most active during slumber.

Next, watch, listen, and feel the meaning of these words in your mind: *I am a patient spirit.*

You may have begun the day as an anxious human. Tonight you will end it as a wise and patient spirit. Feel these words for fifteen minutes. After that, you may fall asleep or continue in a very relaxed state of mind. This is such a critical practice within the art of healing oneself. As patience moves through your body, your life and dreams will change. These days, patience is so grossly underrated. Patient means present. Patience is consciousness. When a person runs around all day, she runs around in her dreams quite unconsciously.

As you give yourself the gift of patient dreaming, you add to the meaning to your life. The greater your self-awareness, the more easily your attitude can heal your body. If you endow your spirit with patience and stillness through the night, your body will heal much faster. Focusing on a patient spirit also holds the key to becoming self-aware or lucid in your dreams. I suggest that you continue to practice patience in your dreams if this happens to you. Flying in your dreams may be an option; however, continuing to build stillness, patience, and self-awareness should always be your top evolutionary priority.

Over the years, I have found several safe and highly effective methods to improve my clients' sleep quality, and my own as well. Of the numerous ways to accomplish this, I have discovered four methods that provide the most calmness, slowness, and relaxation during the night and during the subsequent day. These methods tend to have the greatest number of side benefits, also. They make up my consistent "go to" routines for deeper sleep as of the publication of this book.

EARPLUGGED FOOT SOAKS WITH COLLOIDAL GOLD, FRANKINCENSE, AND MYRRH

Tonight, we are about to get biblical on your feet.

Frankincense and myrrh harbor remarkable, instant anti-inflammatory effects. I have seen frankincense and myrrh foot soaks help soothe gout, arthritis, foot fungus, and warts. Myrrh acts as a wonderful preservative as well. A foot bath that includes myrrh will remain strong for about two days.

Myrrh and colloidal gold have a well-known, relaxing effect on the mind. Colloidal gold in particular proves valuable for enhancing the dream state and providing deeper, softer rest.

Sleep forms the second level in the holistic health pyramid. I believe the three wise men brought gold, frankincense, and myrrh to the baby Jesus because they knew of their strong effects upon mental well-being and physical restoration. After all, they could have brought Yeshua Ben Joseph anything, couldn't they?

You may soak your feet for twenty minutes in a tub filled up to your ankles with pure cold or hot water. You may use moderate amounts of both frankincense and myrrh. Use less than a teaspoon of colloidal gold in your foot bath. A little tends to go a very long way.

When combined with earplugs and a short routine of slow, limbic breathing, this late-night foot bath can do everything short of divine miracles. Sweet dreams!

CHLORELLA POWDER AND TULSI ENEMA

Nearly all manner of physical diseases start in the colon. Why? The colon is our largest waste disposal organ. You can imagine what your room would smell like if you never once took out your trash.

Too often, regaining health is simply a matter of relieving the body of its huge, toxic burden. Almost any kind of comprehensive detox will help the average person fall asleep and gain a sense of calmness. But I recommend you try the chlorella powder and tulsi tea enema if you intend to cleanse your colon, especially if you have difficulty falling asleep. Tulsi tea is renowned for its natural sedative effect, and chlorella powder is a highly nutrient-dense substance. Filling your enema bucket by combining them together, even in very small doses, can do wonders for your body if you get to bed soon after. You will multiply its benefits *fivefold* if you do not eat anything before rest.

Here's the recipe: Use one teaspoon of chlorella and one warm cup of tulsi tea with purified water.

SHEA BUTTER ON EXTREMITIES WITH ACTIVATED CHARCOAL

This simple, classic technique deserves much more popularity. Applying shea butter to your arms and legs will improve blood circulation and deliver essential fatty acids into the skin and muscle. Shea butter's vegetable fats have a wonderfully calming, restorative effect that can help get you—and stay—asleep. Adding activated charcoal to shea butter will assist the detoxification process and draw impurities out of your skin.

Apply a small amount of shea butter with activated charcoal to your arms, the back and front of your neck, and your legs tonight, and observe how much more restorative your sleep can be.

HYDROGEN PEROXIDE, EPSOM SALT, LAVENDER OIL, ROSE OIL, JASMINE, AND COLLOIDAL GOLD BATH WITH PASSIONFLOWER TEA

This is one for the fast movers. At night, steep a cup of passionflower tea while filling a tub for a hot, deeply cleansing hydrogen peroxide and Epsom salt bath. You should use one-third cup of good old-fashioned hydrogen peroxide and one-half cup of Epsom salts. After you have soaked your body for ten minutes, you may add rose oil and lavender oil to make your bath more soothing and enjoyable. If you would like to add even more gentleness, add two drops of jasmine oil and one-half teaspoon of colloidal gold after fifteen minutes.

Try not to fall asleep in the bath. Your bathing should last no longer than twenty minutes. Enjoy!

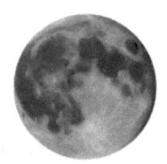

#2 Health Fundamental: Sleeping

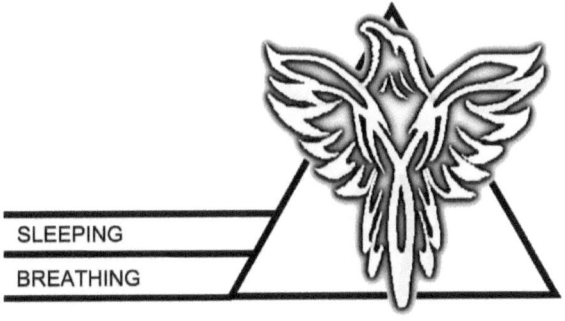

SLEEPING

BREATHING

Although sleep forms the second fundamental on the holistic health pyramid, people tend to take it for granted because most of us have forgotten the magic of true restfulness. Remember, breathing and attitude serve as the primary determinants of great rest.

You would benefit from walking barefoot outside one day (having soaked your feet in olive oil or sesame oil) and lying down on the grass for twenty minutes. While you're grounded, practice a few slow breathing techniques. This has been my daily practice for well over two years. I usually enjoy a nice barefoot walk in the grass. During winter, I use a soft, grounded carpet. This simple action has made a profound difference in my life. The walk has given me a sense of peace, security, sanctuary. Each day, I learn more about energy, slowness, and healing. I insist that you try it and have a pleasant rest.

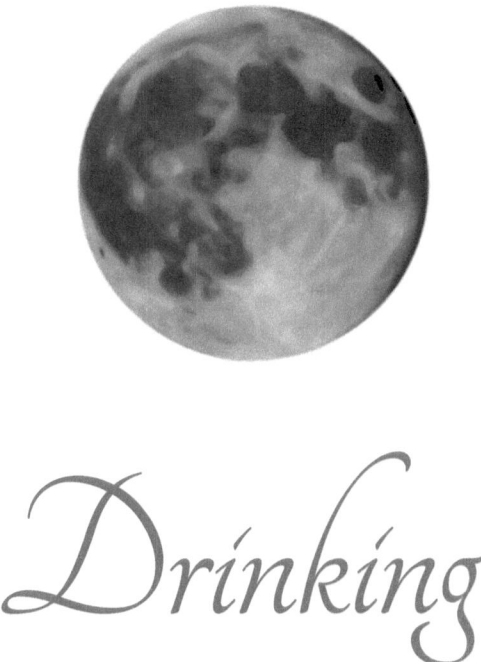

Drinking

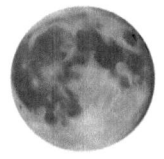

Do You Drink Until You Are Full?

Most people eat until they feel full. That is why I regularly ask my clients, "When was the last time you felt full… on water? Or green vegetable juice?" I almost never get the response, "This morning after I drank my daily glass of fresh lemon water I felt full after my thirty-two-ounce smoothie of protein powder, flax seed, liquid magnesium, and green vegetable juice." That is the answer I seek.

If you have had high blood pressure, heart disease, obesity, depression, stress and anxiety, or cancer, ask yourself first, "When was the last time I snacked on water or had a healthy liquid meal?" I have seen water therapy help heal most of these conditions.

Some experts say nearly 70 percent of Americans are chronically dehydrated. Perhaps dehydration is a hidden epidemic? Amazingly, you can measure people's thirst by measuring the percentage of water of their bodies using an electric impedance scale.

Here is the reality. Several international experts have predicted that within the next twenty years, we will be unable to fulfill the fresh water needs for nine billion people. Already, dehydration is the primary killer of children in the world. That is why I suggest you purchase three separate water filters for your home.

Water vibrates on an infrared spectrum, a frequency level higher than solid mass. This is why water picks up impulses from the human brain, as well as other electrical generators. For more information on water's ability to receive and store psychic information, discover the work of Masaru Emoto.

ACTIVATING YOUR WATER BODY

If I could tell you about the most adaptable, flexible person I know—a special human being who is never rigid in any sense of the word, a friend of mine who gives to ten thousand things and does not strive, who listens to everyone and takes everything in stride—that would be my friend water. Have you met each other?

Water certainly embodies those virtues we seek on our journeys toward peace and stillness. These days, it seems everybody is hot on the path to activating his or her light body. But to activate a light body, you must first discover it. Pure water acts as an excellent magnifier of light. One fresh glass could help.

For the last three years, I have pursued the activation of my "water body." It's been a fascinating quest. I've been drinking, meditating, blessing my beverages, saying fantastic things like, "I forgive you, water," practicing the liquid virtues of equanimity, selflessness, transparency, and so on. It has gone well. I have made numerous discoveries.

Activating your water body starts when you begin to realize that over 70 percent of your body should be liquid, and that with each breath you take, you spur the inner tides of your body.

So let's imagine for a moment that you are lying down, taking long, slow breaths. You are alone in a tranquil setting. You feel the movements of your inner ocean with each inhale. Literally, you feel them. I call this process "mental liquefaction."

Continue just as you were, taking long, slow breaths, immersing yourself in the liquid of you. Focus only on your own liquidity, as well as its movement. Should you lose focus at any time, inhale quickly and exhale through your mouth. This will shift energy to your brain and refocus your attention. In less than twenty minutes, you should find yourself immersed in a deeper brain wave pattern, a brain wave pattern that equates to the high frequency of water itself. If you are new to this type of meditation, you may perform it in a hot, herbal bath.

In this deeper, conscious state, you can either begin your own meditation or fall asleep. Mental liquefaction will bring you into deeper resonance with energy and consciousness, allowing you to heal yourself.

FLUID TIDES OF DNA

A steam pressure system, or a vapor system, fuels the energy in the cells of our bodies. Insufficient amounts of water will block chemical and energy reactions. Even our DNA, swimming in this hot spring of human life, is subject to change.

On DNA and its interplay with its surrounding liquid environment, author Stefi Weisburd cites in her research that "…changes in the environment of DNA such as temperature, acidity, salt level, and water content can drive transformations between these DNA structures…When the mode softens, the amplitude of the vibrations [of the DNA] grows so large that the original structure is destabilized and the molecule is driven into a new geometry."

This means that our DNA is constantly moving, breathing, and dancing in its own water. This must be beautiful to observe. Also, it is one reason I recommend you drink eight to sixteen glasses of water per day.

THE ART OF TOASTING

Human beings verbally bless their water prior to consuming it because water is highly receptive to mental energy. The electrical transmitter/generator in your head is constantly fueled by water. It makes some sense that its receivers would be watery as well. This is what Masaru Emoto has discovered.

Therefore, the art of toasting proves an ideal way to alter the molecular structure of your water, to heal your body, drink slowly, thoughtfully, and discover what you want out of life.

When you toast with red wine and impassioned words, one single taste can have a pronounced effect on your life and body. Modern society practices the art of toasting shamefully backward. You control your sobriety, your mind, your reality. Therefore, toasting is a profound, declarative action. For thousands of years, modest amounts of red wine have helped to drop the veil of fear and limitation.

Red wine is known for its antioxidant content. It has always been used for ceremonial toasting. Red wine has certain beneficial effects on the human nervous system. However, most of them have yet to be scientifically validated. Used righteously, red wine can help purge the spirit better than any drug, psychedelic mushroom, vine, or tea. Toasting ceremonies are traditionally done with fierce passion during sunset. Done properly, two glasses are all you need to make a positive shift in consciousness.

Your words encapsulate who you are as well as who you desire to become. Each word you say has the potential to cast away illusion, doubt, and fear. The eyes might be windows to the soul, but your words create the pathway toward your future. You are crafting that new life through your pronouncement. The most powerful and influential book of the last two thousand years begins with that fabled declaration, "In the beginning was the Word." Jesus Christ once said "Of what I do, you can do greater. Truly, I tell you, if you have faith as small as a grain of mustard seed you can say to this mountain, 'Move mountain', and it will move". I believe your words and message are bonded to your life in a very profound and mystical way. A toasting ceremony done righteously will have people screaming with passion, convulsing with laughter, or weeping with joy after one or two glasses. I have seen this happen. Allow it to be a transcendental experience for you.

Toasting is not for immature people who cannot control addiction; it requires healthy intentions and strong maturity.

"To your health, longevity, and many years of love, peace, and joy."

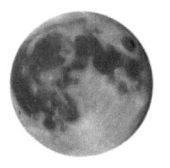

#3 *Health Fundamental: Drinking*

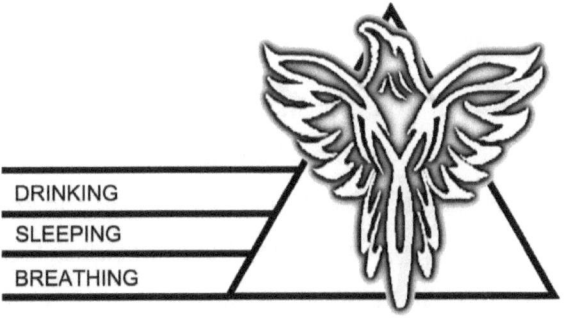

DRINKING
SLEEPING
BREATHING

THE PHOENIX INSTITUTE'S SLOW-DOWN TONIC

2 liters of distilled water

3 tablespoons of whole flax seed

3 tablespoons of powdered kelp

3 tablespoons of spirulina

2 teaspoons of liquid magnesium

1 sprig of sage
1 teaspoon of nettles

Optional:

3 tablespoons of pure plant protein powder
3 servings of dandelion, spinach, cabbage, or kale

Instructions: Blend well and serve

Keep in mind, you do not need to drink red wine to experience a shift in consciousness. By all means, you may enjoy my slow-down tonic. This is a recipe loaded with magnesium, organic sodium, essential fatty acids, and many other calming nutrients. It is a first-class tonic for relaxation and will help still the mind.

If you are allergic to pollen, cat or dog dander, or wheat, this tonic will also provide relief from your symptoms. It's a simple, powerful recipe. So let me to propose a toast!

"Doubt thou the stars are fire; Doubt that the sun doth move; Doubt truth to be a liar; But never doubt I love."
– William Shakespeare

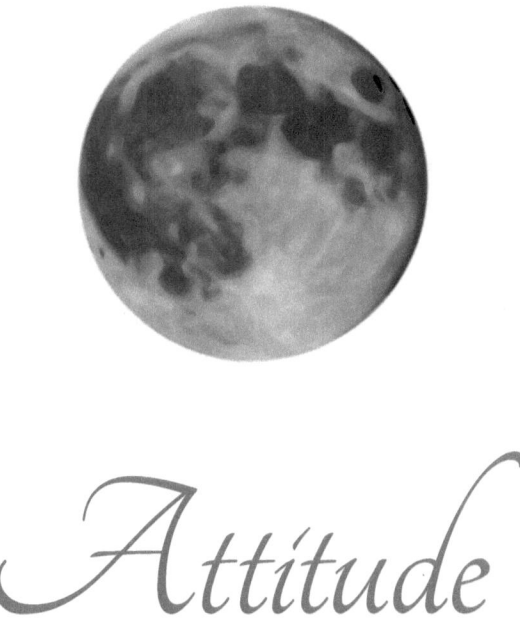

Attitude

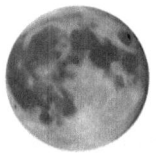

Enter The Void

"Invisible threads are the strongest ties."–Friedrich Nietzsche

During sunset, the ancient Egyptian civilization observed the Law of the Pharaoh. This law suggested that every person hold themselves utterly responsible for their own emotional health. The Law of the Pharaoh decreed that each knowledgeable Egyptian meditate, contemplate, or complete the inner works needed to clear their heart and mind before resting. Ancient Egyptian history spanned over three thousand years. For the greater good of society, perhaps no more perfect law exists than the Law of the Pharaoh, a law now lost to the ages.

Alas, meditation is a lost art. You need not live in China, India, or Egypt to begin your personal practice of meditation, nor must you follow anybody's rules in the process of self-discovery. I have seriously studied transcendental meditation on my own for several years. I would like to humbly offer some personal insight.

Imagine your heart placed on a balance scale, with a tiny feather on the opposite side. Before each night, or perhaps throughout the day, you should weigh your heart against this metaphorical feather. If your heart feels lighter than a feather, or equivalent to the weight of air itself, consider yourself spiritually clear and present. How do we accomplish this? Start by observing all the invisible, inner sources of your suffering. Place them on your scale. Would you like to feel burdened by the woes of your life? Or, would you rather a tiny feather weigh them down?

THE OBJECTIVE AND SUBJECTIVE

One of the most widely recognized transcendental states is the state of nothingness (also termed "stillness," "emptiness," "presence," "eternity," or "love"). I believe they all mean the same thing. These words represent an objective viewpoint that I call "the void." If you find your mind stuck in the past, what better medicine than eternity? If you find your mind stuck on people, places, things, or events, what better medicine than focusing on something devoid of all form? If you feel your mind moving too erratically, what greater kinesthetic medicine exists than a few soothing moments of stillness? Stillness, the void, love, timelessness, and nothingness may all equate to that tiny feather. Innate feelings of love and joy should never necessitate weight, measure, or form. Would you agree? Would you like your problems to weigh you down? Or would you like your problems to be weighed down by a feather? Are your inner demons worth giving up? Ask yourself this question.

As a matter of fact, we know these states of being but often use different names for them because we tend to think in the subjective tense. Words or phrases like patience, trance, attentiveness, observation, living in the moment, love, or hypnosis all describe a state of unfettered presence. All of these attitudes bring us into unworried, untroubled stillness. Without burdens, the human mind is capable of creating beautiful things. How do we get there?

"Doing nothing is better than being busy doing nothing."—Lao Tzu

UNCONDITIONAL OBSERVATION IS THE VOID

Think about the word "observation." When we observe, we become still and present. Try listening right now. What happened? Did you feel still and present? Did you listen to something? I suggest you try this: Do not look, feel, or listen for anything. Rather, create a continuous attitude of unconditional observation. Persist. Feed this unconditional attitude with your unbiased attention so it may grow beyond the limits of your perception. It takes practice, but you'll find sharpening your focus the greatest reward to a meditative practice. Each moment counts. Don't waste a single one.

The Buddha said, "What we think, we become." Consciousness and energy create the nature of reality. Consider the creative principle of consciousness for a moment. Consciousness conditions things. If we aim to bring resolution to our thinking mind—our conscious-ness—it helps to condition our thinking mind toward unconditionality. Therefore, I suggest you focus on the void regularly. Begin by placing your mind and heart on the scale, deeply analyze what weighs you down, then move into the void unconditionally. It's an ancient teaching.

When we create a state of unconditional observation, our consciousness and viewpoint start to expand. By focusing on the "all and nothing," we also reprioritize our personal problems. Why? It is widely believed that the nothingness (the stillness, the void, the emptiness) forms the essential centerpiece of the lost self. The scale's balance begins to tip when the void becomes more important to you. Therefore, by this action we create a space within that fosters peace.

Regardless of your personality or beliefs, focusing on the void can become a key practice in life. Spending two hours focusing on the nothing does not make you a Buddhist. Eternity is not a philosophy. Stillness and nothingness are not religions. How can someone worship nothing? Presence may be a New Age concept; however, one's experience of it often varies more meaningfully than any written word. You must focus for long periods on the void to make it useful for you—that's the key. Otherwise, it will remain a fragmented, meaningless concept. Do not consider the void merely a concept. It is an unconditional non-thing, remember? It works as antimatter for whatever is the matter with you. It can keep you sailing through rough waters. It's the source of spiritual bliss.

Historically, people have mimicked the void in search of supernatural or divine experiences, going without food, living in caves, blindfolding themselves, becoming celibate, doing away with possessions, and all kinds of other things. Most of the time, these people felt their actions represented an appropriate way of life. They surrendered material attachments to tap the power of the void itself. Sensory deprivation proves a useful tool in uniting with the void; however, it is not required. Possessions may be significant, but more important is how you think about them. Always, success is defined as a progressive shift in attitude.

Ramtha, a brilliant, modern teacher, explains, "Focus on the void. It is where we go to be cleansed. It is all things potentially, no thing materially. It is the basis of creation."

Why don't you try it? Don't focus on any one thing. Be still and focus your attention on the unborn, the unseen, the unnamable, the unconditional quality. Sojourn beyond time and space. As you focus on the nothing, you will dissolve the burdens of your past. It works. Finding stillness in life is a critical part of any spiritual journey, I think. When we integrate the nothing, life will change. Unconditional lightheartedness, graceful support, and a loftier, more expansive viewpoint from which to critique and observe all things will become manifest from this essential practice.

WEIGHING YOUR WORDS

What we say is as important as how we say it. Improving your vocabulary, clarity of thought, and articulation does not necessitate learning a bunch of new words every day, although reading can be helpful. Slow communication is another lost art. These exercises will help teach you how to communicate comfortably and concisely. When you learn to use your communication skills properly, you can refine your message and learn how to speak with personal, authentic authority, no matter what.

Let's review the basics: listening to a storyteller, pausing to breathe, and practicing solitary reading.

LISTENING TO A STORYTELLER

Most of us have a storyteller in the family. If you don't, you may research Lord Buckley, Mike Daisy, Garrison Keillor, or simply Google "great American storytellers" for more exposure. You may also seek out famous speakers, lecturers, or comedians. Pay attention to how the masters open a topic, close a topic, and reinforce a topic or message.

PAUSING TO BREATHE

Pause and breathe right before you speak. Most of the time, if you appear composed and comfortable, people will listen much more intently to your words. Why? A great speaker knows how to lengthen a dramatic pause, or allow their audience a moment of contemplation, as they get centered through a deep long breath. Confident speakers naturally pause to breathe. Contemplate and reflect during these brief pauses yourself. It works.

SOLITARY READING PRACTICE

Bring classic literature into your room and passionately read aloud. This can make for invaluable practice time to improve your poise, pause, articulation, and focus. Reading prose or poetry can also prove inspiring and lift your spirit on a gloomy night.

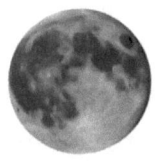

#4 Health Fundamental: Attitude

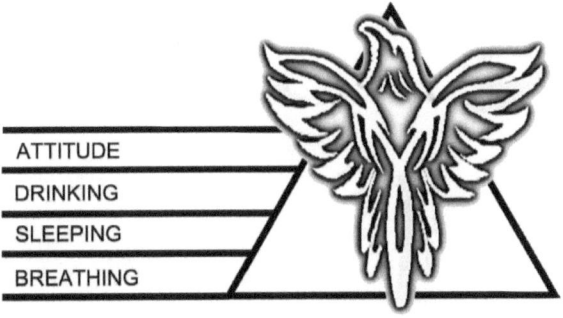

ATTITUDE
DRINKING
SLEEPING
BREATHING

Attempting to craft an attitude of power, understanding, and joy from insecurity and lack proves inspiring work. You should feel proud of yourself. However, often the inner work we do tends to wind us up because parts of our issues remain unresolved due to our lack of either inspiration or knowledge.

True wisdom starts to grow when you can say, "I don't know." When you learn to identify with the unknown and feel at peace among the unknown, the void, the stillness, the eternal, the infinite, you will resolve your fears and start to open new doors into a different understanding.

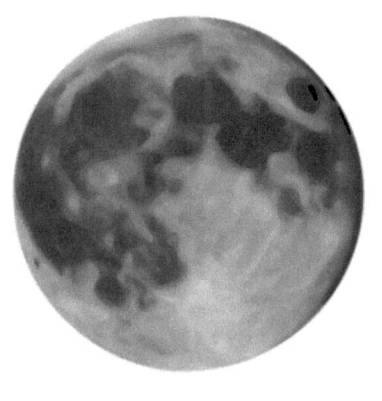

Eating

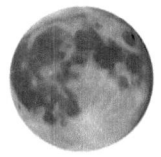

Dietary Corruption

I feel utterly convinced that we could prevent, halt, or reverse most of the health problems in our world today by simply changing our diets. There is a growing concern for the quality of our food in this country. Corporate meddling and government irresponsibility have corrupted common sources of information.

Not so long ago, the *Washington Post*, *Time* Magazine, and the *New York Times* released several articles on organic food almost simultaneously. The authors each claimed that organic foods were as nutritious as conventional farm produce. All of the authors failed to consider the health risks of conventional pesticides, herbicides, fungicides, food preservatives, and other dangerous synthetic chemicals that people consume each day. Nearly half of Americans are overweight, and we are not getting any healthier.

The less chemically coated foods you consume, the healthier you will become. The more food you grow on your own, the healthier you will become. Is it any surprise that the First Family in the White House has elected to eat only local, organic produce?

COOKED AND RAW

You'll find many topics worth discussing when it comes to eating healthily and achieving wholeness. Choosing to eat close to half of your food in the form of organic, clean, raw vegetables will prove a very wise decision. Even wiser, grow your own salads so that when you feel hungry, you can pick your greens, gather your sprouts and seeds, wash them, and eat them straight away. By doing this, you will save yourself energy, time, and money, and perhaps add years to your lifespan. Freshly picked, live vegetables have the potential to create miracles in your life. Personally, I have seen a living food diet help to reverse chronic illnesses in hundreds of people.

However, do not overdo this suggestion. If you consume too many calming foods, you will *suppress* your vitality and energy. That is why it's important to consume a healthy balance of cooked and raw foods. Listen to your body and learn what it needs. Discover your natural appetite mechanism while you focus your intent on achieving wholeness in body and mind.

MASTICATION

The longer you chew your food, the longer you taste your food. Chew raw food for at least forty seconds and cooked food for thirty seconds. Our saliva contains several enzymes that begin digesting our food even as it sits in our mouths. Chewing your food thoroughly will not only aid the process of digestion, it can also strengthen your jaw muscles. Experiment with slow and fast chewing all the time. You will derive much more nutrition from your meals this way.

L- GLUTAMINE, MAGNESIUM, NETTLE HERB, AND B VITAMINS

Generally, I suggest four supplements to help still the mind. L- Glutamine, a B vitamin complex, liquid magnesium, and nettle herb in the form of a tea can do wonders for your body's rhythms.

L-Glutamine serves as a calming brain, bowel, and muscle nutrient that you can ingest with water once or three times a day. It effectively controls sugar cravings, constipation, and headaches, and promotes muscle repair.

Several experts say that over half of the American population is deficient in magnesium, a critical element for improving heart health, healing joints and connective tissues, and relaxing the nervous system.

In the morning, B vitamins can help to detoxify your liver, removing the toxic burden that usually builds up during the night. Moreover, B vitamins tend to promote relaxation and mental clarity, allowing you to just "B". Of all B vitamins, niacinamide and niacin are the most calming. Use niacin in moderation because it causes a strong circulatory 'flush' in the body. Some women may mistake these flushes for hot flashes.

Nettle herb has been used for hundreds of years to improve kidney function, cleanse the blood, remineralize the body, and improve awareness. Several South Americans tribal cultures considered nettle an excellent plant to aid in removing evil spirits from possessed bodies. When combined with chamomile flowers, nettle herb can help relax a very high-strung nervous system.

You may slow yourself down between meals by using any of these four ingredients.

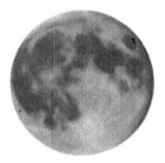

#5 Health Fundamental: Omakase Eating

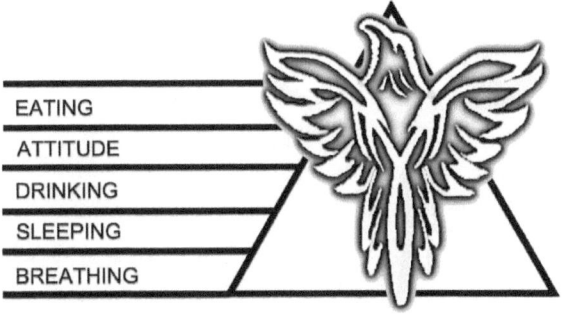

EATING
ATTITUDE
DRINKING
SLEEPING
BREATHING

In Japan, chefs explore the kitchen in an event called *Omakase*. Basically, the chefs can serve up whatever they want for any length of time. People attend such events on the chefs' schedules. *Omakase* can last for hours.

Most Americans would find themselves completely unfamiliar with this wonderful way to eat. Try serving yourself or others in this fashion. You can create memories, spark relaxed conversation, and perhaps develop nice friendships by hosting an *Omakase*-style event.

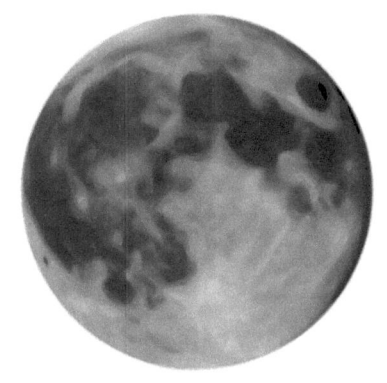

Exercise

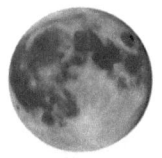

Rhythm Is Exercise And Exercise Is Rhythm

Most people do not exercise on a daily basis because they do not want to feel pain; it's really that simple. Most people who exercise understand its benefit in releasing tension, but very few people enjoy that good, clean rush of energy. Why? Most people attach a mental burden to exercise which, unfortunately, creates physical lethargy. Together, mental lethargy and physical lethargy create a state of health that tends to spiral out of control.

However, exercise comes quite naturally to people who have a good sense of rhythm because they know how to speed up, slow down, and enjoy energy flow. To them, it's all a dance; it's about the journey, not breaking those lethargic barriers of a toxic or overweight physical body. Athletes of rhythm view exercise as an art.

All of the greatest athletes possess superb rhythm. People watch sports because they can freely enjoy the rhythm of a game. People observe the transitions between defense and offense, the crash of a grand slam, the theft of home base, the elegance of a figure skater or a simple Olympic foot race, all without getting out of their own seats. Rhythm resides innately in us all.

As Gabrielle Roth, creator of the 5 Rhythms practice, once said, "You cannot say you don't have any rhythm, because even the words, 'I don't have rhythm' need a sense of rhythm."

People also fail to exercise because they feel burdened and bogged down by pain itself.

THE WINDOW OF PAIN

Pain results from a misappropriation of energy. You can use several methods to relearn effective movement. Yoga, dance, and the Alexander technique can all prove remarkably effective in beginning your reeducation in movement and form.

To begin, sit up straight. Take a deep breath. Now, grab the corner of this page as if you were going to turn it. With the least amount of effort possible, slowly turn the page back and forth a few times. Have you been using more than the required amount of energy to turn these pages? This is what we do all day long. We think too fast, press too hard, and breathe like tiny mammals.

Try drinking a glass of water ever so gently, with the least amount of effort possible. You may find it an excitingly new sensation. Now, try breathing as gently, and as lightly, as possible. Are you getting the picture? Learning to use energy as rhythm is a key that unlocks exercise and health. Turn on a favorite tune and start to dance. Dance lightly at first, without any form, pattern, or restraint. How awesome does this feel? By way of rhythm, our bodies naturally try to right themselves in the correct balance and alignment of energy.

This forms part of the work of Jonathan Horan, Gabrielle Roth, Amara Pagano, Douglas Drummond, Lucia Horan, and many other leaders in the global 5-Rhythms community. I insist that you to check them out soon. You will find the 5 Rhythms practice a liberating and remarkable healing dance that is way ahead of its time.

HIKING

Take a cue from nature: she's always having a "slow day." Hiking is a great way to get in touch with your slow rhythms. The warm biofield of trees, the healthy particulate matter in the air, the soothing and hypnotic sounds of a living forest all provide a golden chance to explore yourself, decompress, and empty your troubled mind.

TAI CHI

You can perform the solitary exercise of tai chi anywhere. It focuses on finding your center point—or center of gravity—as you move your breath, body, energy, and mind in one motion.

SURFING

Though it can take some effort, surfing provides an exciting activity highly conducive to stillness and rhythm. Who could think of a more agreeable environment than an ocean or a beach?

As I have mentioned, water exemplifies the quintessential embodiment of nature's rhythm. While surfing, or rhythmically moving through the shore, you learn about water. Water can allow you to float, sink, dive under whitecaps, or carve your way through huge waves, all while rocking you up and down ever so gently. The ocean has the tendency to open up the lungs, cleanse the skin, and refresh the mind.

GARDENING

When we arrive at the dirt, we form a connection to power plant Mother Earth. Digging in soil, planting a seed or flower, and then tending to it takes a lot of physical labor. Select an excellent location for your garden, conducive to both you and your plants. Will it be close to home? Off in the corner of the yard where it will be undisturbed by children or pets? You can make that choice.

PAINTING, DRAWING, AND TRACING

Painting is an incredible exercise in stillness. Why? It requires that you hold an image utterly still in your mind and then reflect it onto the canvas or paper. Your strongest and most sophisticated "muscles" are in your head. Your brain uses an enormous amount of energy each day. Painting, drawing, or tracing great works of art while remaining still and focused proves a calming task for the busy mind.

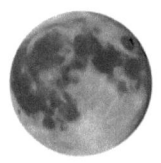

#6 Health Fundamental: Exercise

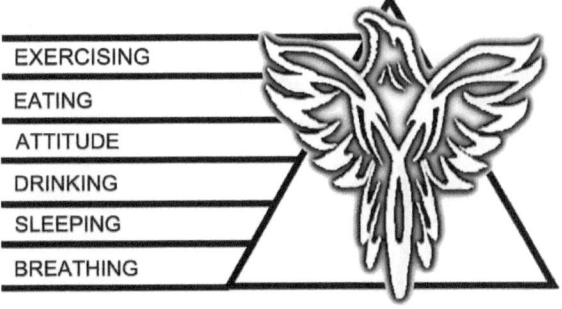

EXERCISING

EATING

ATTITUDE

DRINKING

SLEEPING

BREATHING

Physical pain and inner suffering are like being stuck in a hurricane. If you're outside, you will likely get caught in the rain and wind. If you find shelter, the storm temporarily abates, though it still continues over-head, greatly limiting your mobility. If you examine the wind and its movement, you may begin to form a strategy. Perhaps it is wise to take shelter for a few long moments, but what if the winds and rains never let up? Where will you run?

You can find quiet and peace in the center of the storm. Standing in the eye of a hurricane is an awesome experience. There is no more perfect wisdom than navigating through life in the eye of the storm. The winds blow most powerfully toward the central ring. You will have to constantly build your determination. You will have to stay strong. You will have to know how to use your energy. Learn how to move. Timing is everything.

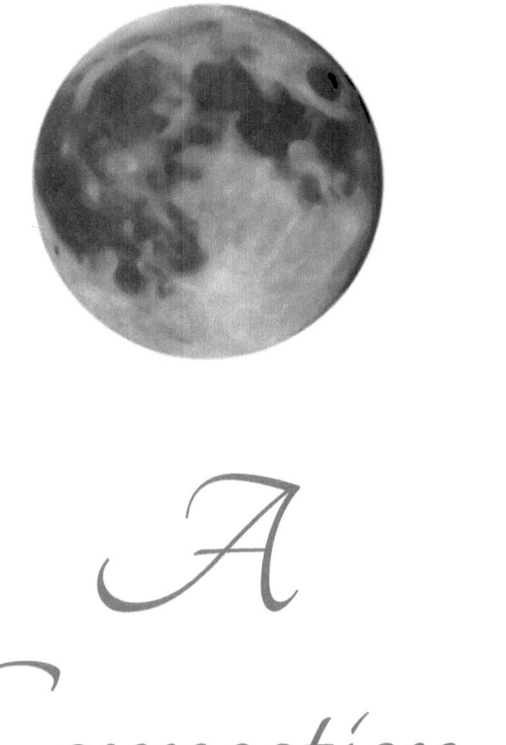

A
Connection
To Nature

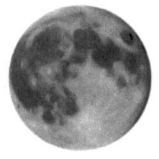

Sweat, Swim, Bonfire

Make the exploration of nature a top priority in your quest for slowness. I highly recommend you become initiated into the rhythms of nature Native-American style. To do this, go online and find a sweat lodge in your local community or out in the country. Make sure that it has a bonfire set up and a nice, cold body of water nearby. An ocean, river, or lake can suffice.

Then take my advice: Go there. Sweat. Get wet. Then get dry. You won't find a more enchanting way to experience the gentle, evolutionary touches of nature.

SLOW LOVE AND MATING

Relationships and relationship problems preoccupy modern society more than anything else. The emotional experiences of them represent the high and low markers in most people's lives. Some people do not know how to be happy unless they have someone in their lives to fill the void. Others are plagued with anger, insecurity, and fear. Still others cannot help but feel victimized in relationships, while some people cannot help but abuse the level of bonding, trust, and communication that forms when two people get to know one another. At the root level, human instinct tells us to master and control those things in life that provide pleasure. During this quest to possess another human being, most find that they, too, would like to be possessed. It is, perhaps, the human condition at its best; however, it is the spiritual condition at its lowest.

There is a difference between living like an animal and operating from the essence of humanity itself. True love resides in the unseen. A love based on the contents of one's character will always outlast the superficial adoration of one's physical structure, financial assets, or survival intelligence. If love can last, it has a chance to grow. If love is real, it must be born slow.

We would all be better off if we studied the mating habits of other animals rather than learning the simplistic functions of sex. Eagles and other raptors are known to mate for life and to defend, and even die for, one another. Dolphins, elephants, and vultures are known to be the most devoted and gentle caregivers of their young. Some raptors and a few species of sea turtles will not find a new mate if they lose their life partners. A few species of lizards mate for life; however, most of them mate spontaneously, and rarely, if ever, do they protect, comfort, or show regard to their mates. A large percentage of animals mate in this fashion. Some animals copulate, live, and care for each other for an indeterminate amount of time, then quarrel with each other and move on.

So love and companionship exist in nature, by varying degrees, and human beings have the inclination to imitate the entire lot, whether lower or higher animals. This is a beautiful thing, because every man and woman has the inalienable right to discover which level of companionship and love serves him or her best. That encapsulates the journey of relationships through life.

In order to facilitate your journey, let us further clarify the definition of sexuality and love according to Mother Nature.

Always, sexuality falls into two categories: male or female. The mating behaviors of males and females are genetically opposite from one another. Passion forms the root attitude of male sexuality. The male is genetically programmed to spread his seed, or ejaculate, as many times a day as physically possible. However, survival forms the root attitude of female sexuality. The female is programmed to foster the continuation of life. In most species, the female gender is the stronger gender for this reason.

Not only is the male disposition opposite from that of the female, the genitalia itself is reversed in form. In the human body, the largest cell is the female ovum and the smallest is the male spermatozoa. Even more startling, the electromagnetic field of the male opposes that of the female. So the next time you look at the opposite gender, remember that you are gazing at your genetic opposite. We are not the same, from an animal perspective.

Love, according to Mother Nature, is much simpler. The giving of life force forms the root attitude of love. Whether the father works his hands to the bone in support of his family, or a soldier sacrifices his or her life on the battlefield, or a babe rests in the arms of a woman, or a spiritual shaman sings to heal the dying, or an eagle defends its mate, or a nursing mother dog suckles stray neighborhood kittens, or the songs of the poet inspire forgiveness and purposeful living, love simply gives life. We are all one and the same from the perspective of an unconditional lover.

What makes human relationships complicated is our breeding, which compels us to fit into civilized gender roles. What makes human relationships so wonderful is that, by virtue of mingling with our opposites, we break civilization's gender roles. If you observe a happy man and a proud woman interacting together, you will grasp the significance of this concept. We are meant to break rules with one another.

Modern gender roles limit humans more than root animal attitudes do. Take the two common, modern archetypes for women, the daughter/mother roles. Historically, society has taught daughters to find wealthy men (survival) and raise their daughters to act in an unselfish manner while often expecting things to be freely given to them. The archetypal mother, meanwhile, is the relentless caregiver, a woman systematically taught to sacrifice her own life force, often without any discernment on her part.

Women trained to sacrifice their power to another hold this entire stratification of gender roles in place. In the male-dominated world, women find it challenging to develop themselves to an equal degree of stewardship, at least insofar as "*his-tory*" can recall. Though women are relegated to a different scope and standard, such women as Queen Victoria, Madam Curie, Susan B. Anthony, and others have made undervalued contributions to humanity. Many powerful, mature women have created lasting contributions to humanity, even while swimming upstream. Albert Einstein once said, "Logic will get you from A to B. Imagination will take you everywhere." A mature woman is a creator by nature, who, when deeply in love with herself, can wield her own power with wisdom. A mature woman can be queen of the chess board, an unconditional lover, and truly a magnificent creative force.

Without self-acknowledgment, self-contemplation, reflection, and a sense of worthiness, the latent love that resides in all women will never be defined, and thus never used properly. Untrained love, lacking definition, is not useful.

As you may have guessed, the two common gender roles for males are the son and the father. Historically, society has taught their sons to be cruel, highly competitive, and completely self-interested, often to the detriment of other men and women. The archetypal father lacks forward vision, is highly predictable, lethargic, rigid, and a reliable provider.

Modern males are systematically taught out of their curiosity, and instilled with tremendous amounts of pressure, responsibility, and fear, usually at a very early age. A mature man is a reliable, poised explorer with an open mind. It only took a handful of male inventors to create the industrial age, mind you. Men are philosophers by nature, with an incredible knack for discerning patterns within environments. Men create definition. They measure the stars. Men like this can provide order and balance to women, and potentially to all people on earth.

The mother philosopher, the father creator, the charitable son, and the visionary daughter all are very rare non-archetypal breeds; however, they do naturally exist. The personal degree of spiritual and natural evolution within them creates a force capable of harmonizing all of modern society.

This is why relationships are so vitally important. Without them, civilization would remain stagnant in its social values, its gender identity, and, in particular, its humaneness. Many of us have mothers who act more like daughters, or fathers who act more like sons. Many people do not know how to change, nor do they even know why they should. That is the folly of life according to modern social conscious thought.

Modern women and men contrast so much, like night and day. So, for males, the journey of an honorable relationship is often fraught with overpowering lust, jealousy, competitiveness, and possession. For females, relationships are often fraught with unworthiness, confusion, and insecurity. A more profound connection to all of life begins when you initially examine your gender opposites, your genetic opposites, your social conscious opposites, and your spiritual opposites. With inner work, the right kind of insight can help you to gain power over your insecurity, your confusion, even your lust. You can be a slave to your human pleasures, or you can learn to master them. Learn all you can about what you need, what you lack, and what you already have as a man or woman. One day, when you learn to hold yourself in unity, above social consciousness, the true alchemy of love will be born within your own soul.

A LIST OF RELEVANT QUESTIONS

If you have made the choice to relate on a level beyond the common herd in an effort to understand your other half, I would recommend that you get to know each other better. Here is a list of questions you may ask each other:

Who makes you laugh more than anyone?

If you could spend a day with anyone in history, from politics, religion, arts, and any other field, whom would you choose?

Tell me about you best friend from childhood.

How long do you think you could go without watching TV?

If you had all the money in the world and could quit your job to work in any field, which field would you chose?

If you could pick your first name, what would it be?

What is the first book you remember reading?

Did you have a childhood idol?

Would you lie to keep your job?

Have you ever been on television? Would you like to be? How would you prefer to be portrayed?

What is the luckiest thing that ever happened to you?

What was the best job you ever had?

Have you ever been on vacation alone?

If you were stranded on a desert island and could only have one thing, what would it be?

Describe the worst date you've ever been on.

Are you a morning person?

What is your earliest memory?

What was the most difficult paycheck you ever earned?

Do you ever wish you had started something much earlier in life?

Have you ever loved anything other than another person?

What was your favorite subject in school?

If you could change sexes for a whole month, tell me what you would do, day by day.

Can you describe your family in four words or less?

What was your favorite Halloween costume?

Do you have a favorite holiday?

If you knew you would die within one year, what would you do?

What is your favorite thing to do that does not cost money?

If you were reincarnated as an animal, which animal would you be?

Do you like looking through family photos?

What is the most embarrassing situation you have ever been in?

Do you like watching any sports?

If you could be an Olympic athlete in any sport, which sport would you choose?

Where would you like to go that you have never been?

What was your proudest moment?

Have you ever lied about your age?

What book has had the most profound effect on you?

Do you believe in astrology?

Do you believe in numerology?

Do you believe in scientology?

Who is your favorite family member?

What possession would you never consent to share?

Have you ever slept outdoors?

Have you ever slept on a beach at night?

How would you like to be "spoiled"?

What qualities do you admire in the opposite sex?

How would you break off a relationship?

Have you won any awards?

Have you ever thought of running for political office?

Who is the most eccentric person you know?

Have you ever thought of becoming a Buddhist monk?

What does the word 'strength' mean to you?

What does the word 'love' mean to you?

When do you find yourself confused?

A BLIND DATE DONE RIGHT

Use these questions on a blindfolded date. You can conduct this date over the telephone, the Internet, or you can take it to the next level and consider meeting in a public park with friends. Have them create a circle around you and your blindfolded date. Remember a few of the questions listed above and remain blindfolded yourself.

No cheating! This is probably the best way to get to know someone. You may consider creating a local blindfolded speed-dating chapter in your community. This could prove a highly entertaining activity for you and your peers. (I urge you not to engage in any blindfolded dinner dates, because it is difficult to use utensils while blindfolded.)

BEING COMFORTABLE AND SOCIABLE

In order to facilitate your slow love and mating process, you must make friends with the opposite gender. If you do not have anyone in your life, a friend of the opposite gender can help keep you comfortable and interested in the opposite sex. If you feel nervous when meeting with the opposite gender, friends such as these are treasures, provided you work to keep them strictly as friends. This may seem difficult, but it is important to see the long-term value in these friendships and not toss them aside for what you want in the moment.

Very often you will find it useful to begin these friend-ships by stating outright, "I need help feeling comfort-able around women (or men). I honestly find you easy to relate to, and I want to be your friend."

Speed dating is also a wonderful way to purge your first-impression jitters. Try meeting sixty new people in ninety minutes. Learning how to speak and what to tell people within the first five minutes of meeting them will prove a useful life skill. Speed dating also provides skills for those looking to make a good impression on job interviews or acting auditions. Many people prac-tice their acting prowess through speed-dating events.

Lastly, free dancing is an absolutely superb way to break down your inner rigidities. I recommend taking your platonic friends and your mate to the 5 Rhythms prac-tice. Dancing your heart out with people you love can add powerful meaning and substance to even a very dull life. Your body will thank you, and your spirit will be pleased.

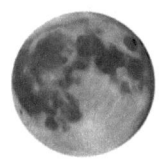

#7 Health Fundamental - A Connection to Nature- Breathing

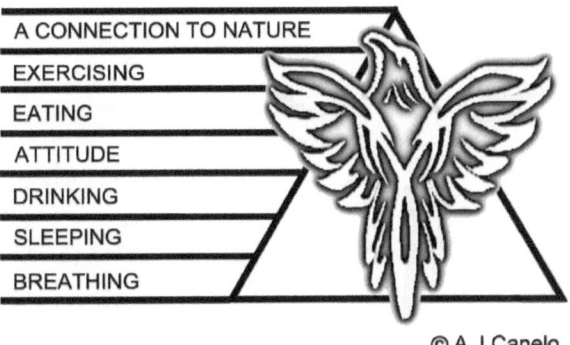

A CONNECTION TO NATURE
EXERCISING
EATING
ATTITUDE
DRINKING
SLEEPING
BREATHING

© A.J.Canelo

"THE PEAKS OF LIFE"

Stillness is elevating. Tonight, if you live in the country, go out and explore the highest terrain you can find. If you live in the city, discover a very tall building with an open roof. Go up there and bring this book with you.

Try a few breathing exercises on this remarkable high point. Observe the night.

From a loftier perspective, you can easily observe the push and pull of life, its struggle and its rhythms, the promise of a new day.

Standing there, alone or with a friend, find peace inside. Let the wind dry your tears. Move your heart. Free your mind and let loose your soul. You may not live a life of cascading stillness, wholesome peace, tranquility, or love. However, this moment deserves to live apart from the shadows of time.

I think we will all get there someday. Rest well.

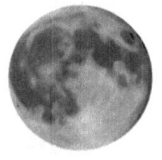

Take The Pyramid Author's Challenge

If you are a young doctor or health coach aspiring to write a book, I offer you this challenge.

Write a manuscript of at least sixty pages reinterpreting my holistic health pyramid from your perspective. Your topics may include, but are certainly not limited to, women's health, hormone health, health futures, health history, environmental awareness, autobiographical interpretations, health messages in story form, global health, community health, spiritual wholeness and health, addiction, longevity, or combinations thereof. You must display the holistic health pyramid in its original form on the back cover of your book. Electronic books will be accepted.

The deadline for this project is May 25, 2015. All who submit manuscripts to me will be mentioned in my later books. I will select three winners. For each winner, I will write an introduction for your book. For the second place writer, I will donate five hundred dollars to help you begin publishing or self-publishing your book. For the first place writer I will donate five hundred dollars to your publishing, as well as offer you a chance to accompany me as a guest speaker to one or more annual health fairs and festivals.

We all have a story in our pyramid. I would love to read yours. Help me share the magic of the holistic health pyramid while you seize the opportunity to enhance your career, writing talents, and personal education.

All the best,

Anthony James Canelo

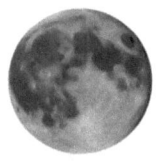

Thank you so much for your inspiration, encouragement, and support:

Emily Canelo, Peter Canelo, Nicholas Canelo, Cheryl Stoll-Thygerson, Charles Walters, Jeff Baker, Justin Baker, Russell Ditchfield Agboe, Christina Devilla, Dr. Majid Ali, Dr. Brian Clement, Dr. Kazim Mirza, Eric Levinson, Peter Frisa, Kristen Boyer, Andrew Wertheimer, Paul Mantel, Matthew Mantel, Avery Mantel, Viktoras Kulvinskas, Ryan Monay, Theodore Nathan, Rebecca Bullón, Osayuwame Olijah, Monique Lussier, Gail Barnett, Lucia Rose Horan, Andrew Goor, Monica Day, Matthew Chambers, Ramtha, and JZ Knight.

The 5 Rhythms dance community of New York City WBAI 99.5 FM New York City and their listenership, and the NDNS family.